Weight Loss Epiphany

The Workbook

Angie J. Hernandez, C.Ht.

Disclaimer

The Publisher and the Author make no representations or warranties with respect to the accuracy or completeness of the contents of this work and specifically disclaim all warranties, including without limitation, warranties of fitness for a particular purpose. No warranty may be created or extended by sales or promotional materials. The advice and strategies contained herein may not be suitable for every situation or person. This work is sold with the understanding that the Publisher is not engaged in rendering legal, accounting, medical, health or other professional services. If professional assistance is required, the services of a competent professional person should be sought. Neither the Publisher nor the Authors shall be liable for damages arising herefrom. The fact that an organization or website is referred to in this work as a citation and /or a potential source of further information does not mean that the Author or the Publisher endorse the information, the organization or website may provide or recommendations it may make. Further, readers should be aware that internet websites listed in this work may have changed or disappeared between when this work was written and when it is read.

To Gamal, my biggest supporter.

Because you believed in me, I could believe in myself.

- Angie

TABLE OF CONTENTS

Introduction to Weight Loss Epiphany

Welcome, to Weight Loss Epiphany, the Workbook. Weight Loss Epiphany is an effective way to change the way you look and eat food. You will also find this workbook will help you change the way you think and speak to yourself, internally. Changing our judgemental thinking about ourselves, is key when making life changes around food. What you'll love is how easy this is.

Resolve, right now, to take responsibility to complete the exercises and follow the instructions to the letter and success will be yours.

I've included exercises and homework which includes the recordings of the Weight Loss Epiphany sessions and HypnoMeditations, sold separately. You will find listening to the recordings relaxing and pleasurable, making these lifestyle changes possibly the easiest changes you've ever made.

Assignment Number One

You've embarked on a life change today and just by sitting down with this workbook, you're well past the first few steps of your journey. This is a program to lose weight or release weight, as I like to say, but it's not only that.

This is also a journey of self -discovery. We don't just eat to fuel our bodies, we have emotional attachments to food. Learning more about ourselves while improving our health is a life bonus.

In this first assignment, you will:

1. Define Your Goal

2. Create Your Own Goals

3. Swiss Cheese Your Motivation

4. Calculate your future weight for an upcoming event.

5. Picture yourself at your goal weight

6. Receive your week one homework assignment.

1) Define Your Goal

You might wonder about the purpose of a written assignment, after all, you bought the program, isn't that enough to turn your bad habits around?

Your Subconscious Mind relates to the world through all of its senses; touch, sight, sound, smell, and taste. When you only engage part of the senses, you limit your chances of success.

In the Weight Loss Epiphany Program, you will be appealing to all five senses whenever possible. The persons that find the most long-term success with this program, are those that embrace each part of it wholly.

Writing is an important part of success because handwriting is a learned response leading the information right into your Subconscious Mind.

To define your goal, follow these guidelines:

1) Use only positive statements stated in the present tense. Eliminate words such as : no, not, won't, don't, can't, try or want. These simply blow up that statement in your mind, making it gain in strength. (Don't think of a giant purple banana! Of course, now, that's all you can think of!)

So, if you want to stop eating junky foods; avoid saying, "I want to stop eating junk food." Instead, state the positive way you'll be eating, "I eat fruits, vegetables and lean protein each day."

If you want to curb your portions, choose positive wording like, "I can feel satisfied with small, very filling amounts."

If you plan to exercise often, you might say it like this, "I take recess three times a week and I love it!"

Write below, three positive statements about your weight release outcome.

1)

_____

_____

_____

2)

_____

_____

_____

3)

_____

_____

_____

2) Create Your Own Goals

No one but you can create your own future. You are in charge and in control. Make your goals centered around your behaviors, habits and feelings, You can't control what others do, you can only control yourself.

So, when writing your goals, avoid the behavior of others such as, "My spouse eats the same meals as I." or "I hear compliments every day.". Make it about you. "I eat healthy and nutritious foods daily." "I plan out my meals a week in advance." "I have an emergency meal plan, just in case.

List three goals here, centered around your feelings and behavior.

1)

_____

_____

_____

2)

_____

_____

_____

3)

_____

_____

_____

3) Swiss Cheese Your Motivation

How do you eat an elephant? One bite at a time!

If your goal seems huge and daunting, then it's too big. Swiss cheese it! Take out little holes one at a time and before you know it, you've hit a milestone.

So, set yourself an attainable goal that adds up to a bigger goal down the road.

Instead of thinking, "Two pounds a week will not be enough. I'll still be fat!", try thinking this way, "Losing two pounds a week is the safe and steady way to go. At that rate, I'll be twenty-four pounds slimmer in three months. Won't I look good in some new clothes?!"

Write out one Swiss Cheese Goal:.

_____

_____

_____

_____

4) Calculate Your Future Weight for an Upcoming Event

Now that you've defined your goal, it's time to give your mind a treat. A little glimpse of the future that will motivate your mind to support you on your way.

Think of an event a few weeks our from now. It could be a party, a class reunion or maybe just the start of the golf season but choose an event and figure your weight loss for that day.

Here's how to do it:

Most people average a five pound loss the first week on this program. After that most lose one to two pounds per week. So, if your event is six weeks from now, you would calculate your loss like this :

Week 1 = 5 pounds lost

Week 2 = 2 pounds lost

Week 3 = 2 pounds lost

Week 4 = 2 pounds lost

Week 5 = 2 pounds lost

Week 6 = 2 pounds lost

15 pounds total lost

You can estimate losing fifteen pounds over the next six weeks.

Now, go out this week and buy a new piece of clothing that will fit you when you have released fifteen pounds. This piece of clothing is a Vision Board for your subconscious mind. Hang it in a spot where you'll see it each morning and each evening before sleep. It's important that it's new. It needn't be expensive. It can be a Tee shirt or a belt; a blouse or a pair of shorts. But, make it something new for you to fit in at the time of your event.

Calculate your weight loss for your event.

Week 1 = _____ pounds

Week 2 = _____ pounds *Add more weeks, if you need to.*

Week 3 = _____ pounds

Week 4 = _____ pounds

Week 5 = _____ pounds

Week 6 = _____ pounds

5) Picture Yourself at Your Goal Weight

Now, and in the future, I want you to picture yourself at your goal weight. I had a hard time with this myself. But I learned there are a couple of ways to do it.

You can picture yourself at a younger age when you looked slimmer. Pull out an old picture of yourself and tape it here or out where you can see it. Keep that body in your mind and allow your mind to pull you to it like a magnet!

Another way to accomplish picturing your slimmer self, is to find an image of someone you consider to have the size you desire and print out their picture. Try to make it someone of similar height and body type. Now, put your head on the body in the picture! It might sound funny but your subconscious mind doesn't know the difference and will pull you toward that image.

Put your ideal image here:

_____

_____

6) Week One Homework

A) Weight Yourself

Post your start weight here _____

(Only weigh yourself once per week)

B) Take body measurements

(Measure yourself once per month)

Take your measurements and note them here.

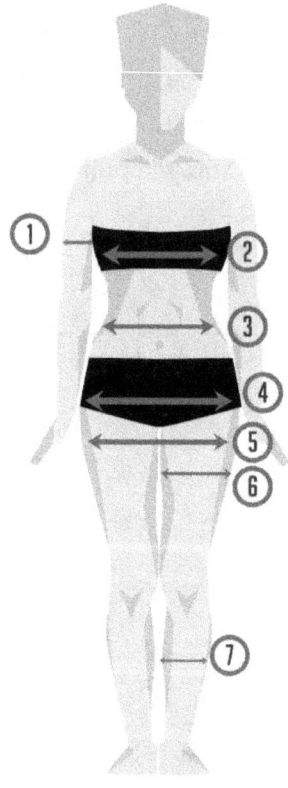

1) Upper Arm _____

2) Bust _____

3) Waist _____

4) Hips _____

5) Thighs _____

6) Upper Thigh _____

7) Calf _____

C) Learn Tapping on my Website, *www.IndianaHypnosisCenter.com*, so that you can use the bonus HypnoMeditation recordings each week.

D) Listen to Session One, Weight Loss Epiphany, at least once a day (before dinner is a good time).

E) Listen to your HypnoMeditation for Weight Loss once a day.

This week's affirmation: I will vent out what is holding me back from losing weight, in early morning dreams.

Assignment Number Two

Welcome to Session Two! You've made it through your first seven days of Weight Loss Epiphany! Aren't you surprised how easy it was? You can be so proud of yourself for what you've accomplished.

It's time to weight in again and you can post your current weight here:

Last week's weight:_____

Today's weight:_____

Wow, you are doing so well and I'm proud of you for making it to this point.

This week we'll be setting new goals to help you along the way and creating a challenge, as well. I want to see if you're up to it. You know you are.

We'll be covering these points:

1) Walking challenge.

2) Read the Four Key Ingredients to Weight Loss Success

3) Show off and hang your new piece of clothing.

4) Explain Slim and Fir Thinking vs. Fat Thinking

5) Receive you Week Two homework assignment.

1) The Walking Challenge

This week I'd like to challenge you to walk 10,000 steps daily. This is an easy way to kick start your fitness. You probably already walk in your everyday life at home and at work. But now you'll be able to see just how much you do and challenge yourself to do more.

To give you an idea of how 10,000 steps balances out, 2000 steps is about one mile. And in 1/2 hour, the average person walks about 3000 steps. So, when you put in 10,000 steps, you are putting in about a five mile walk.

Now, I understand that you could be in a situation where walking five miles is not up to your current physical ability. I recommend that you touch base with your doctor about your fitness level.

You can use an alternative workout in this case; like Tai Chi, swimming, Yoga or isometric exercises and stretching. The idea is to get moving in some way.

For most of you, walking is a good exercise. I suggest you download a free App to your phone to measure your walking. Go to the App Store you prefer and type in "pedometer". You will see a selection. Choose the one that most appeals to you.

Post the number of steps you've walked this week here:

Walking Chart

> Sun. | Tues. | Wed. | Thurs. | Fri. | Sat

Number of step ____|_____|_____|_____|____|____

2) The Four Keys to Weight Loss Success

A) Truthfulness - At this turning point in your life, it's time to take a good look at yourself and face the music. How do I feel about where I am? How did I get here? It might be time to admit your own responsibility about your situation. Look at yourself and take charge of your life. Ask yourself why do you do the things you do?

B) Responsibility - It's time to and also important to look at where you are and take responsibility to make change. This is not about assigning blame. It's about recognizing that you have control and show you're willing to take charge and make changes, a little at a time. Move yourself into a better place; mentally, physically and spiritually.

C) Commitment - Take that commitment you already have toward your family, pets, children, job, friends and causes and add yourself into that same category. It's time to make yourself just as important as your kids, your relationship and your job! Pledge to yourself and take it seriously. You are worthy of your care and you deserve it. Take your life back!

D) Inner Strength - You're going to face challenges but, even though it might not be easy, you will get through with inner strength, understanding and determination. You will need patience to learn to understand and empathize with yourself. But overcoming each challenge, increases that self-esteem and motivation. Once you overcome one hurdle, the next one is a little easier. Hypnosis can and will increase this inner strength and motivation from within. Each step on this journey makes you stronger and more determined in your goal; a healthier, happier life.

You deserve to love yourself enough to improve your health.

3) Show off and hang your new piece of clothing

By now you've purchased your new piece of clothing. Write a description of it here.

_____

_____

Good, now hang your clothing in a spot where you will see it when falling asleep and waking in the morning. This is the Golden Half Hour. That time when you are naturally in hypnosis. Since your subconscious mind is open at this time, it will look at this piece of clothing, recognize it's purpose and work hard to draw you to it. That means your subconscious mind "sees" your purpose of releasing weight and steps up to the plate; helping you make your way into that clothing!

Along with your new clothing, hang that image of your slimmer self that you created this week with it. Draw your subconscious to the new you and the new clothing. Isn't this exciting?

4) Slim and Fit Thinking vs. Fat Thinking

Did you ever wonder why some people seem to go through life, facing food easily and keeping their size with little effort? At the same time, some of us struggle with our size and worry over what we eat; making each bite seemingly "bad" or "good".

That's because some people have Slim and Trim Thinking and others have Fat Thinking. Let me explain what I mean.

Slim and Trim Thinking people do not treat their emotions with food. Fat Thinking people eat when they're anxious, sad, upset and even when they're happy and celebrating. Slim and Trim Thinkers might even stop eating when their emotions are high. They might say, "I'm just too upset to eat!" Slim and Trim Thinkers find other ways to handle stress like talking it out with a friend, soaking in a bubble bath or going for a run, They might prefer to take action like looking up information and formulating a plan. Fat Thinkers use food to distract themselves from the upset. The upset is still there but, for a little while, they are eating it away. The problem is that later, Fat Thinkers regret the eating and are disappointed in themselves compounding the problem.

Overweight persons can be drawn to food through external cues like ads on TV, pictures of food on social media, seeing another person eating, smelling food or thinking of a person who used to cook for them. Slim and Trim people eat from internal cues. They might notice a feeling in their stomach, they might be yawning or feel fuzzy, or their mouth might be wanting that certain flavor. They might even drink a full glass of water before indulging, just to see if they were thirsty and not hungry.

Fat Thinking people eat <u>until</u> ... they might eat until their plate is clean, eat very quickly, eat past the time when they feel satisfied, wolf down their food while absorbed in TV or the computer or their phone. Slim and Trim Thinking people will pause after each few bites and take stock. When they feel satisfied, they stop eating, no matter how good it tastes. They just reject that hard stomach feeling that overeating makes.

Fat Thinking people attach emotion to their food. "This cookie is calling my name." "Chocolate is my downfall." "I can't resist potato chips." "I need my comfort food." But to Slim and Trim Thinkers, this is ridiculous. To them, food is just something you use when hungry, otherwise, no big deal. Even when the food is tasty, Slim and Trim thinkers can be satisfied on a taste or a couple of bites. After all, it's the first two bites of any food that tastes the best, right?

Fat Thinkers use denial when their weight creeps up. They often stay away from the scale because seeing the numbers brings them down. This can really send your weight out of control. Slim and Trim Thinkers use the scales as a tool. When their weight fluctuates more than two to three pounds, they make changes right away to bring it in line.

List three things you can do to handle your stress other than eating.

1)

_____

_____

_____

2)

_____

_____

_____

3)

_____

_____

_____

What do you say about your food when you feel a craving? It's calling my name, it's my friend, I have to have it...? Write that here.

_____

_____

Now, write down the opposite of the statement you wrote above. For example, you might write: "Chocolate is my friend.".

Now write a truer statement:" A friend doesn't make you fat or overeat. Chocolate is just something I crave when what I really need is to stretch and relax from stress for a few minutes."

_____

_____

_____

5) Week Two Homework

A) Post your weight loss here. _____

B) Listen to Session Two, Finding Satisfaction, at least once a day.

C) Listen to your HypnoMeditation for Safety in Weight Loss, once a day.

D) Use your Slim and Trim Thinking.

This week's affirmation: I release old ideas about good and respect all my body does for me.

Assignment Number Three

Welcome to Session Three! By now you're hitting your stride and feeling pretty great about yourself! You can be proud of your progress and I'll bet the realization is coming to you, that this is the easiest program you've ever been on. Won't it be easy to continue through your life eating three small meals a day?

Weigh in again and chart your loss here:

Last week's weight _____

This week's weight_____

Loss this week_____

Loss last week_____

Total_____!

This week we're meeting new challenges with a one-two punch!

We'll be covering these points:

1. Re-cap 10,000 steps progress

2. Write a Self-Image paragraph

3. Learn self-hypnosis

4. Receive you Week Three homework assignment

1) Re-cap Your Walking Challenge

Your challenge was to work on walking 1,000 steps per day using a pedometer or a pedometer app.

If that was too hard a challenge for your physical ability or your doctor recommended an alternative physical workout, then rate your exercise choice appropriately. List the time limit of your workout or the number of times you fulfilled your goal. It's all good!

List here how you measured up to the physical challenge this week and how you plan to move your body this coming week.

Number of steps this week _____

Alternative workout: number of times you exercised_____ or duration of workout_____

My workout goal this week is_____

2) Write a Self Image Paragraph

This is a description of who you are, but you're not writing about the Present Moment You, you are writing about Future You who is Slim and Fit. What we will do here, is write about the Future You but say it in the present tense.

Let me show you what I mean. Your Future Self will be as a slim and fit person; a big change from the person you started out as when we began Weight Loss Epiphany. So, the Future You might be described something like this in your mind:

"I will wear size ten clothing. I will look in the mirror then and like what I see. My son will hug me and say, "I can reach all the way around you now!" I will go on rides at Disneyland and fit in all the seats. People won't look at me that way they do now. I will be proud of myself and not need all the medications I do now."

But we want the Subconscious Mind to buy into our new image and want to take us there. To do that, we need to take out words like "will" and "won't". When you use future tense words like those, the Subconscious Mind completely blows you off. It doesn't believe in some make believe future. The Subconscious Mind only believes in the NOW and is only motivated by now. So, let's go back and re-write that self- image paragraph in the Now!

"I comfortably wear size ten clothing. When I look in the mirror, I like what I see. My son is hugging me, saying, "I can reach all the way around you now!" I am riding at Disneyland on any ride I want and I fit beautifully in any seat. I love how I look and how others admire my fitness. I am proud of myself. My doctor says I don't need all of those medications!"

Write your Self-Image Paragraph:

_____

_____

_____

_____

3) Learn Self-Hypnosis

Self-hypnosis is easy and practical. You can learn it here but the lesson will last you a lifetime. You don't need to use it more than a few minutes a day but the change you can make in your life can be profound.

Here is how you do it in a few easy steps:

a) Find the blank template at the end of this chapter. Use it to formulate your self-hypnosis sessions, as many as you choose. You are in charge.

Spell out the problem you wish to address, then plan it on your template. (Use the enclosed examples as your guide.)

b) Slip into hypnosis. You've been practicing with the recorded sessions and now you can do it on your own. There are many ways, such as focusing on a spot on the wall, counting yourself down from five to zero (deep sleep) or flexing and relaxing your muscle groups one at a time. Come into that state of focused attention.

c) Focus on the solution to your problem thinking over how your will think, feel and act.

d) Imagine, picture or pretend that you are carrying out the new behavior. This is called a Mental Rehearsal.

e) State positive affirmations so that you can remind yourself about creating this change you want.

f) Now, craft your own post-hypnotic suggestion like this:

From now on, when I encounter (this) _____, I (do this) _____.

g) Come up and out: open your eyes, count yourself up from zero to five and give a big stretch.

That's all there is to it! I've made some examples to get you started and they are all using a strong commitment to change. Your commitment to change should look like this:

• focussed on the positive

• using your own strengths

• contain statements that rely on what you think, what you feel, and what you say and what you do

• all about the solution, not problem based

• always based in the future

• focussed on your own actions, not depending on anyone else or something outside of you to happen

• specific. This solution should occur at a certain time and place where you implement your solution. When (this) happens, I (do this). Stay away from vague thinking like, I want to be happier.

• use all your senses. Your words and what you visualize, even what you smell, have big effects on your Subconscious Mind.

Take the blank template and make as many copies as you need . Use them to frame a problem then design your own solution for it. Use these steps and then take yourself into a light state of hypnosis, concentrating on creating your solution. After that, count yourself up and out. Use only a few minutes and soon you will be able to move through self-hypnosis quickly and easil

If you choose, you can also record your own voice reading out the hypnosis session to use later. You might prefer having the recording to just listen to and concentrate on. In this case, you fill in the template, then use your device or phone to record your self-hypnosis session. Have fun with it and use all the wording and positive reinforcement you can.

Sample Self-Hypnosis Template One *by Judith Pearson, PhD*

1) Describe your problem or concern. _I eat whenever I feel stressed out.   Example: whenever someone criticizes me._

   _____

2) Self-hypnosis induction. Take three deep breathes and count yourself down.

3) Create the solution: what is your new response? How will you think, act and feel?

   New thinking: _Criticism is only another person's opinion. It is not necessarily accurate. I_ can treat it just as information that may or may not be useful to me.

New feeling: I detach from the criticism so that I can remain objective about it.

New actions: I respond calmly and tactfully.

4) Visualize yourself carrying out this new action in a situation that previously would have been challenging. This is your mental rehearsal.

I visualize a co-worker criticizing one of my reports, saying things I feel are unfair. I take a deep breath and feel relaxed. I tell myself that the criticism is only information for me to evaluate. I feel calm and detached I calmly look at the co-worker and say, "I'll gladly listen to any specific recommendations for improvement."

5) Your positive affirmations. The calmer I feel, the more I make wise choices about food. I am in charge of my own self-esteem, and no one else can take it away from me. I eat only when I feel

hungry. When I feel stressed, seek solutions not more food!

6) Your post-hypnotic suggestion:

From now on, whenever I encounter someone criticizing me, I calmly take a deep breath and recall that I am in charge of my self-esteem and feelings. I think clearly and remind myself that I am okay and criticism is only information. I respond calmly and tactfully. I feel good about it afterwards.

Bring yourself up and out. Count up from zero to five, give a big stretch and take a deep breath. You're done!

Sample Self-Hypnosis Template Two *by Judith Pearson, PhD*

1) Describe your problem or concern. I need to exercise more often.

2) Self-hypnosis induction. Take three deep breathes and count yourself down.

3) Create the solution: what is your new response? How will you think, act and feel?

New thinking: I know exercise makes me feel great physically, emotionally and mentally.

New feeling: I feel motivated to exercise. I anticipate it, look forward to it.

New actions: I schedule a regular time for exercise and I do it!

4) Visualize yourself carrying out this new action in a situation that previously would have been challenging. This is your mental rehearsal.

I am in my workout clothes. I am smiling and moving and using my muscles and breathing heavily. I am sweating happily and giving my body a good workout. I pace myself. I make exercise fun by listening to music or doing it with a friend. I stick with my routine and honor my exercise time. I feel fantastic afterward. I see the results as my conditioning, energy and stamina improve.

5) Your positive affirmations. Exercise makes me strong and healthy. Exercise helps me tone my body, manage stress, build endurance and increase my personal power. I enjoy movement and stretching. I am a physical being and my body was made to move. I stay fit and firm! I experience the grace and beauty of a healthy body and a healthy mind. When it comes to my workout, there are NO EXCUSES!

6) Your post-hypnotic suggestion:

From now on, whenever I encounter my scheduled workout time. I suit up, feeling powerful and excited. I take deep breaths and stretch. As I begin my workout, I move at my own pace. As I continue, I feel happy about my increasing strength and flexibility. Even sweat and heavy breathing tell me I am doing something good for myself! I feel pride that I am taking care of my body in this

way. I continue to move through my routine,
giving myself encouragement to go on. Is I cool
down, I feel satisfaction with my effort. Afterwards,
I feel great, and my entire day seems to go
better.

7) Bring yourself up and out. Count up from zero to
five, give a big stretch and take a deep breath.
You're done!

Self-Hypnosis Template *by Judith Pearson, PhD*

1) Describe your problem or concern.

_____

_____

_____

2) Self-hypnosis induction. Take three deep
breathes and count yourself down.

3) Create the solution: what is your new response?
How will you think, act and feel?

   New thinking:

_____

_____

_____

New feeling:

_____

_____

_____

New actions:

_____

_____

_____

4) Visualize yourself carrying out this new action in a situation that previously would have been challenging. This is your mental rehearsal.

_____

_____

_____

Your positive affirmations.

_____

_____

_____

5) Your post-hypnotic suggestion:

From now on, whenever I encounter

_____

_____

_____

Bring yourself up and out. Count up from zero to five, give a big stretch and take a deep breath. You're done!

4) Week Three Homework

A) Weigh In

B) Listen to Session Three Recording, "New Path", at least once a day.

C) Listen and participate in your HypnoMeditation, "Tapping for Clarity" once a day.

D) Write out a solution to a problem on your Self-Hypnosis Template and use self-hypnosis to implement your plan.

This Week's Affirmation:

My confidence rises each day and encouragement seems to appear in my mind, as I were my own best friend.

Assignment Four

Congratulations, you've made it to Session Four, Dreaming into Success! You have successfully made this way of eating a habit that can take you into a new vision for the rest of your life. You may have been struggling for a long time with your weight or it might be something that cropped up as new to you after having a baby or changing jobs or a trauma that happened. No matter what caused you to gain weight, now you know how to release it. You don't even have to struggle like so many do. You don't have to give up lists of your favorite foods. It's just that easy.

Now it's time to finish this part of your journey of discovery. You aren't done. You're only just beginning. This is the way to eat from here on out. Even though you won't have more workbook chapters to work on, this is not the end of your insights into your own self-motivation. Using the recordings daily to reinforce the habit, using self-hypnosis to overcome bumps in the road, and changing your self talk to present tense and positive affirmations, is the way to make all the rest of the changes you choose to make in your life. It's the way to keep this way of eating and thinking a permanent habit.

Let's take a moment to weight in:

Last week's weight_____

This week's weight_____

Loss this week_____

Now, let's see the overall loss

Starting weight_____

Ending weight_____

You can be proud of yourself! You've made huge strides! It isn't all about the scales either. Changing your habits around food is very hard and you've done it! You've impressed yourself by doing something impressive!

In this fourth assignment, you will:

1. Learn the Four R's and put them into practice.

2. File a Personal Injury Suit against Perfectionism

3. Write a Thank You Note

4. Have a Talk from Your Old Self

5. Receive your last homework assignment

1) Learn the Four R's

It's time to put a stop to all the negative self-talk that you say to yourself all day long. It's like a tape that runs on a loop in your head all day long. And, boy, are we mean to ourselves! We've practiced talking to ourselves in the present tense and eliminating negatives. Now, let's get down to the nitty gritty and blast that mean stuff completely out of our head.

- **Reframing**: Maybe you say things to yourself that are mean but you think you need to be mean or you will never reform. Has that really helped you make meaningful changes so far? You don't need to cut yourself down to discipline yourself. Maybe the intent behind the words is positive. So, let's just rephrase it so it is inspiring rather than intimidating. Because, I don't know about you, but I tend to rebel against anything that tries to intimidate me.

  Like this: you might think, "I'm too dumb to learn to dance (swim, Pilates, yoga, Tai Chi or whatever) for exercise." The intent behind this is positive, you want to exercise in a new way but you don't want to look foolish. So we *reframe* the wording so it is positive and supportive. " I find new ways to exercise that are fun. I learn these new ways with other beginners so we are all in the same stage of learning."Maybe you will feel more confident if you come into something new with a little practice. "I find new ways to exercise that are fun and I take a few lessons on YouTube first to get the hang of it."

Rewrite one of the old messages you play in your head and reframe it to the positive.

_____

_____

- **Refuting**: When you say something silly and just mean to yourself, just convince yourself that it isn't true. Give yourself evidence and don't take the criticism. For example you might say to yourself, "I'll never meet my goal. It's too hard." Don't take that kind of talk! Remember just what's on the line; your self-worth.

  Refute it with evidence: "I don't believe any statement that says 'never' because that's just an exaggeration. I've faced many hard things in my life and I came through those. I can do this, too. It's not even close to as hard as those times were. I'm a lot tougher than I seem."

  Refute something you always seem to tell yourself.

  _____

  _____

  _____

- **Refusal**: Don't allow yourself to listen to the negatives. When you hear a put down in your head, whether it's your voice or someone else's, just stop and say to yourself," No! I refuse to listen to this stuff. I don't deserve it and I would never talk like this to my child or even my pet! I certainly won't take it from my own self!"

Imagine that your mind is like a television. If you don't like a show, you change the channel. So, if you hear the crappy talk; change the channel!

- **Replacement**: consciously stop yourself and replace the negative talk with a positive; right away! It's hard at first but in a very short time you'll find yourself doing it on autopilot.

You know so many of us find it hard to say, "I love and accept myself, respecting my body and my mind.". But we have no problem thinking, "I'll always be fat and I just can't change that." This is Stuck Thinking and it leads to unhealthy patterns of behavior. Your subconscious is listening and it will carry out your negative orders. So, order up some of the good life instead!

2) A Personal Injury Suit against Perfectionism

Are you tough on yourself always holding yourself to a standard higher than anyone else? At the end of the day, do you always think about all the things you didn't do? Maybe you're a perfectionist.

Trying to always be perfect is a standard none of us can live up to. If you think you have to be perfect, you'll be disappointed every day of your life. I think you should sue yourself for pain and suffering damages! It's terrible to live each day feeling you're not good enough and never measuring up to your own imagination.

Eating is no way to escape self criticism. I suggest that instead of trying to be perfect, and failing each day, you should shoot for Excellence. Isn't Excellence an awesome standard to live by? And Excellence is attainable and certainly a worthy goal to achieve for anyone. You have a margin of error with Excellence that we need as humans.

List a couple of ways you can allow yourself to be human as well as Excellent.

_____

_____

_____

_____

3) A Thank You Note

It's high time you wrote a thank you note to your body. It might not be perfect or look the way you want it to yet. It might feel like sometimes the two of you are in a battle. But that's not true. Your Subconscious Mind directs your body to protect you at all costs and it takes the information you feed it to do this. It uses all of your senses, sight, smell, touch, taste and hearing, to take in messages and allow your body to react accordingly. It also takes into account your memories and self-talk as a guide in how to behave and protect yourself.

For the whole of your life, your body has done its best to heal you when you're hurt, to pump in strength when you're threatened, to alert you when it needs maintenance and to save up for hard times. And how do you show your gratitude? Well, using this program, Weight Loss Epiphany, is one way to reward your body and mind with positive improvement in your thoughts and actions. But let's give credit where credit is due. Even though you've done your darndest to overlook the messages from your body about what it needs; like "I'm full, I need to move more, I need more rest and sleep, I can't function on alcohol alone", your body still found ways to recover and keep you going. So, let's acknowledge all your body does for you and promise to listen to the signals your body gives you, a little better.

Dear Body,

_____

_____

_____

4) A Talk From Your Old Self

This is the place where we write a note to our Future Self who is slim and fit. Write to that person who will look at this a year from now. Give your future self some advice about continuing this healthy lifestyle you've begun.

Dear Self,

_____

_____

_____

_____

5) Your last homework assignment

a) Weigh in _____

b) Take you monthly body measurements.

_____

_____

How many inches have you released?

_____

c) Listen to your recording for this week and your HypnoMeditation at least once a day.

d) Practice self-hypnosis twice this week.

It has been my privilege to be your guide on this Weight Loss Epiphany. I'm proud of your progress and I would like to hear from you about it! You can contact me at www.IndianaHypnosisCenter.com or on Facebook, Angie J. Hernandez, Certified Hypnotherapist. My hope for you is a life of continued joy and a happy relationship with yourself.

For in person sessions call Angie J. Hernandez, C.Ht. at (574) 658-4686.